THE ANTI-INFLAMMATORY DIET FOR NEWLY DIAGNOSED

Eating Your Way to a Healthier Body and Mind

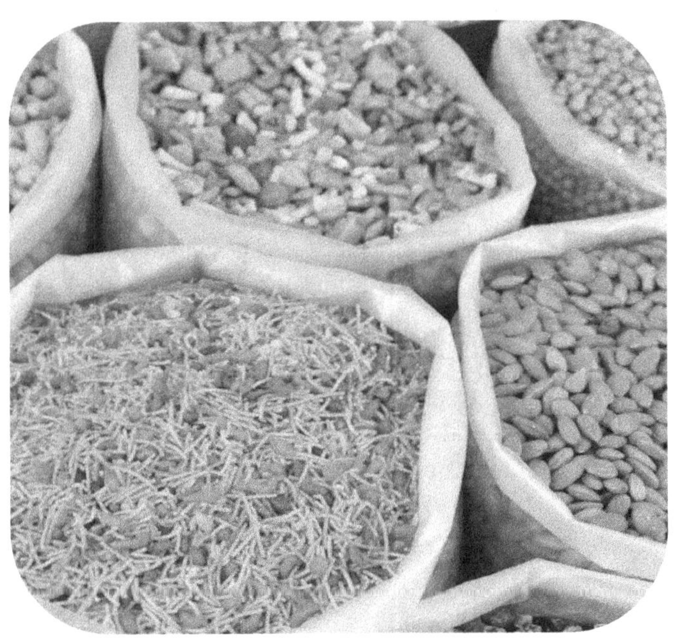

Doc. Joe G Clark

Copyright © 2024 **by Doc .Joe G Clark**

All rights reserved. No part of this publication may be reproduced, distributed, or transmitted in any form or by any means, including photocopying, recording, or other electronic or mechanical methods, without the prior written permission of the publisher, except in the case of brief quotations embodied in critical reviews and certain other non-commercial uses permitted by copyright law.

This book is a work of nonfiction. The views and opinions expressed in this book are solely those of the author and do not necessarily reflect the official policy or position of any organization mentioned. The author and publisher have made every effort to ensure the accuracy of the information herein, but errors and omissions may occur. Readers should consult with a professional where appropriate

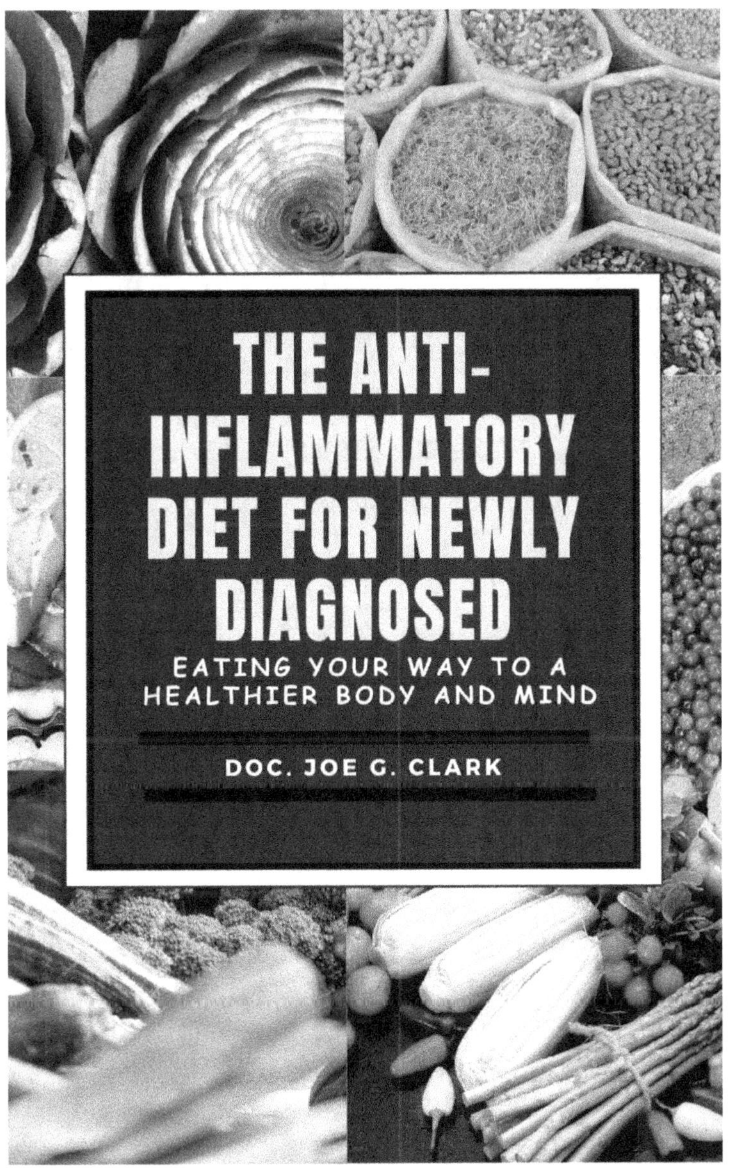

THE ANTI-INFLAMMATORY DIET FOR NEWLY DIAGNOSED
EATING YOUR WAY TO A HEALTHIER BODY AND MIND
DOC. JOE G. CLARK

Table of contents

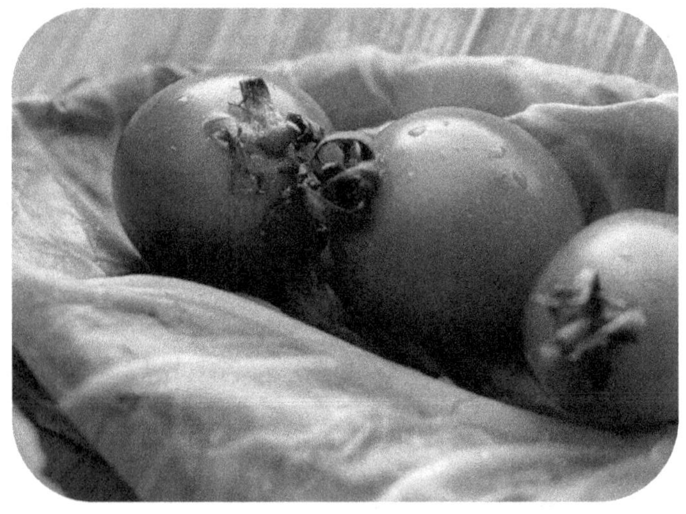

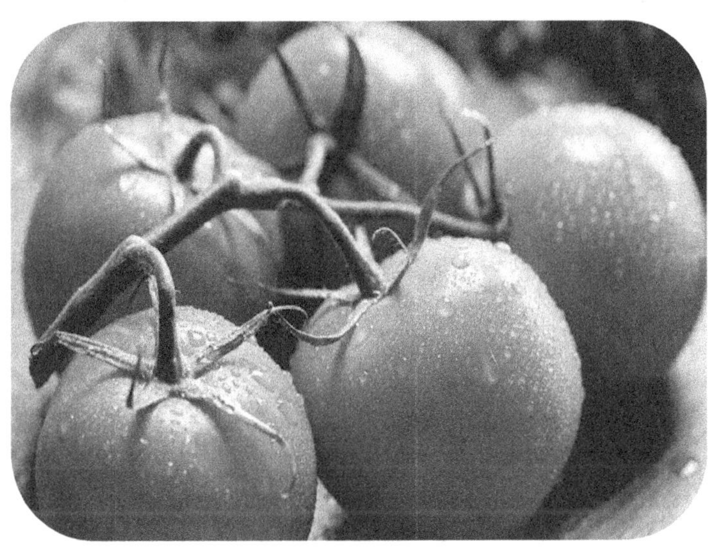

INTRODUCTION

Welcome to **"The Anti-Inflammatory Diet for Newly Diagnosed: How to Eat Your Way to a Healthier Body and Mind."** If you've recently been diagnosed with a condition that involves inflammation, whether it's arthritis, autoimmune disease, or another health concern, this book is designed to be your guide to navigating the world of nutrition to support your healing journey.

Inflammation is a natural response by the body to injury or infection, but when it becomes chronic, it can wreak havoc on your health. Chronic inflammation has been linked to a wide range of diseases, including heart disease, diabetes, Alzheimer's, and certain types of cancer. Fortunately, one of the most powerful tools we have for combating inflammation is right at our fingertips: our diet.

The anti-inflammatory diet is not a fad or a quick-fix solution. It's a way of eating that focuses on consuming whole, nutrient-rich foods that have been shown to help reduce inflammation in the body. By making thoughtful choices about what you eat, you can not only manage your symptoms but also promote overall health and well-being.

In this book, we'll explore the fundamentals of the anti-inflammatory diet, including what inflammation is, how it affects your body, and why certain foods can either exacerbate or alleviate inflammation. You'll learn practical tips for stocking your kitchen, planning and preparing delicious meals, and navigating social situations while adhering to your dietary goals.

We'll also delve into the importance of exercise, stress management, and sleep in managing inflammation, because true health is about more than just what you put on your plate. Throughout the book, you'll find actionable advice, delicious recipes, and strategies for staying motivated on your journey to better health.

Whether you're just starting out on your anti-inflammatory diet or looking for fresh inspiration and guidance, this book is here to support you every step of the way. Remember, healing is a journey, and with the right tools and knowledge, you have the power to transform your health and reclaim your vitality. Let's get started.

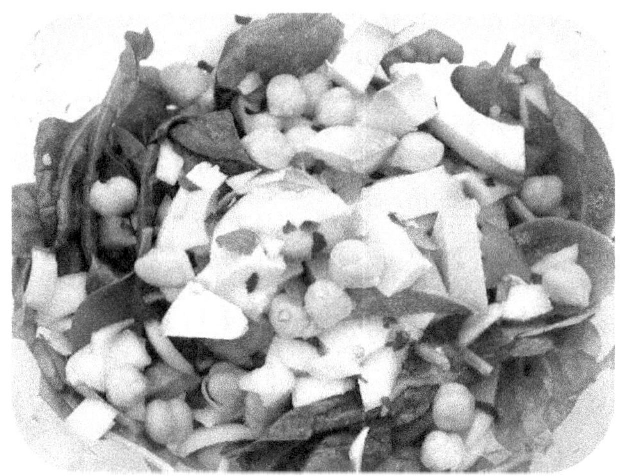

CHAPTER 1: UNDERSTANDING INFLAMMATION

Inflammation is a fundamental physiological response by the body to injury, infection, or irritation. It is a complex process involving various cells, chemicals, and signaling pathways, all working together to protect the body and facilitate healing. While acute inflammation is a necessary and beneficial part of the body's defense mechanism, chronic inflammation can have detrimental effects on overall health and contribute to the development of various diseases.

What is Inflammation?

Inflammation is the body's immediate response to harmful stimuli, such as pathogens, damaged cells, or irritants. When tissues are injured or infected, the immune system is triggered to initiate an inflammatory response. This response is characterized by a series of events aimed at isolating and eliminating the injurious agent, removing damaged tissue, and initiating the healing process.

Key features of inflammation include:

• Skin reddening and warmth as a result of increased blood flow to the region.

• Leakage of fluid and immune cells from blood vessels into surrounding tissues, resulting in swelling.

• Activation of immune cells, such as white blood cells and macrophages, to identify and neutralize pathogens or foreign substances.

• Release of inflammatory mediators, including cytokines, chemokine, and prostaglandins, which help coordinate the immune response and promote tissue repair.

Acute inflammation typically resolves once the underlying cause has been addressed, allowing the body to return to a state of equilibrium. However, when inflammation persists for an extended period, it can become chronic and contribute to the development of various health problems.

The Role of Inflammation in Disease

Inflammation plays a central role in the pathogenesis of numerous diseases, ranging from autoimmune disorders to cardiovascular conditions. While acute inflammation serves as a protective mechanism, chronic inflammation can have widespread systemic effects and contribute to tissue damage, organ dysfunction, and disease progression.

Among the many health issues linked to persistent inflammation are:

• Rheumatoid arthritis and other autoimmune disorders: In these conditions, the immune system mistakenly attacks healthy tissues, leading to chronic inflammation and joint damage.

• Cardiovascular diseases: Chronic inflammation within the blood vessels can promote the formation of plaques, narrowing the arteries and increasing the risk of heart attacks and strokes.

• Type 2 diabetes: Inflammation is believed to play a role in insulin resistance, a hallmark feature of type 2 diabetes, as well as complications such as neuropathy and nephropathy.

• Inflammatory bowel disease (IBD): Conditions such as Crohn's disease and ulcerative colitis involve chronic inflammation of the gastrointestinal tract, leading to symptoms such as abdominal pain, diarrhea, and bowel damage.

• Neurodegenerative diseases: Chronic inflammation in the brain has been implicated in the pathogenesis of Alzheimer's disease, Parkinson's disease, and other neurodegenerative disorders.

Understanding the role of inflammation in disease is essential for developing strategies to prevent, manage, and treat these conditions effectively. By targeting inflammation through lifestyle modifications, including diet and exercise, it may be possible to mitigate symptoms, improve outcomes, and enhance overall quality of life.

Chronic Inflammation: Causes and Effects

Multiple factors can contribute to the development of chronic inflammation, such as:

• Persistent infections: Chronic infections, such as viral hepatitis or periodontal disease, can trigger ongoing inflammation within the body.

• Autoimmune disorders: Conditions in which the immune system mistakenly attacks healthy tissues can lead to chronic inflammation and tissue damage.

• Environmental factors: Exposure to environmental pollutants, toxins, or allergens can provoke chronic inflammation and contribute to the development of respiratory, skin, or other inflammatory conditions.

• Lifestyle factors: Poor dietary choices, sedentary behavior, chronic stress, and inadequate sleep can all promote inflammation and increase the risk of chronic disease.

The effects of chronic inflammation extend beyond localized tissue damage and can impact multiple organ systems throughout the body. Chronic inflammation has been linked to:

• **Accelerated aging**: Persistent inflammation can accelerate cellular aging and contribute to the development of age-related diseases.

• **Immune dysregulation**: Chronic inflammation can disrupt normal immune function, leading to increased susceptibility to infections and impaired wound healing.

• **Metabolic dysfunction**: Inflammation has been implicated in the pathogenesis of obesity, insulin resistance, and metabolic syndrome, all of which increase the risk of cardiovascular disease and type 2 diabetes.

• **Neurological impairment**: Chronic inflammation in the brain has been associated with cognitive decline, mood disorders, and neurodegenerative diseases.

By addressing the underlying causes of chronic inflammation and adopting anti-inflammatory lifestyle habits, it may be possible to reduce inflammation, alleviate symptoms, and improve overall health outcomes. In the following chapters, we will explore the principles of the anti-inflammatory diet and lifestyle, providing practical strategies for managing inflammation and promoting optimal well-being.

CHAPTER 2

The Basics of the Anti-Inflammatory Diet Principles of the Anti-Inflammatory Diet Foods to Include Foods to Avoid Importance of Balance and Moderation

THE BASICS OF THE ANTI-INFLAMMATORY DIET

The anti-inflammatory diet is a way of eating that focuses on consuming foods that are rich in nutrients and have been shown to help reduce inflammation in the body. By incorporating these foods into your diet while minimizing or avoiding those that promote inflammation, you can support your body's natural healing processes and promote overall health and well-being.

Principles of the Anti-Inflammatory Diet

The anti-inflammatory diet is based on several key principles:

1. Emphasize whole, nutrient-dense foods: Focus on consuming a variety of whole foods that are rich in vitamins, minerals, antioxidants, and phytonutrients. These include fruits, vegetables, whole grains, nuts, seeds, and legumes, which provide essential nutrients and have anti-inflammatory properties.

2. Prioritize omega-3 fatty acids: Omega-3 fatty acids, found in fatty fish (such as salmon, mackerel, and sardines), flaxseeds, chia seeds, walnuts, and hemp seeds, have potent anti-inflammatory effects. Aim to include sources of omega-3s in your diet regularly to help reduce inflammation and support heart and brain health.

3. Limit omega-6 fatty acids: While omega-6 fatty acids are essential for health, excessive consumption of omega-6-rich oils, such as corn, soybean, and sunflower oil, can promote inflammation when consumed in excess. Aim to reduce your intake of processed foods and cooking oils high in omega-6 fatty acids, opting instead for sources of healthier fats like olive oil, avocado, and nuts.

4. Choose lean protein sources: Include lean sources of protein, such as poultry, fish, tofu, tempeh, and legumes, in your diet while minimizing consumption of red and processed meats. Plant-based protein sources are particularly beneficial as they contain fiber and phytonutrients that have anti-inflammatory properties.

5. Incorporate anti-inflammatory herbs and spices: Herbs and spices like turmeric, ginger, garlic, cinnamon, and rosemary have powerful anti-inflammatory properties. Incorporate these flavorful ingredients into your meals to enhance both taste and health benefits.

6. Opt for whole grains: Choose whole grains such as quinoa, brown rice, oats, barley, and bulgur over refined grains like white rice and white flour products. Whole grains are rich in fiber, vitamins, and minerals, and have been shown to help reduce inflammation and lower the risk of chronic diseases.

Foods to Include

• Fruits: Berries, citrus fruits, apples, grapes, and cherries

• Vegetables: Leafy greens, broccoli, cauliflower, carrots, sweet potatoes, and bell peppers

Fish high in fat: mackerel, trout, salmon, and sardines

• Nuts and seeds: hemp, walnut, flax, chia, and almond seeds

• Legumes: Beans, lentils, chickpeas, and peas

• Whole grains: Quinoa, brown rice, oats, barley, and bulgur

• Various healthful fats, including nuts, seeds, avocados, and olive oil

• Spices and herbs: rosemary, cinnamon, ginger, garlic, and turmeric

Foods to Avoid

• **Processed foods:** Highly processed foods, including fast food, packaged snacks, sugary drinks, and refined grains, often contain unhealthy fats, added sugars, and artificial additives that can promote inflammation.

• **Trans fats:** Avoid foods containing trans fats, such as margarine, fried foods, and commercially baked goods, as they have been shown to promote inflammation and increase the risk of heart disease.

• **Excessive sugar:** Minimize consumption of foods and beverages high in added sugars, such as candy, soda, pastries, and sweetened cereals, as they can contribute to inflammation and metabolic dysfunction.

• **Red and processed meats:** Limit intake of red meat (beef, pork, lamb) and processed meats (bacon, sausage, hot dogs), as they have been linked to inflammation, cardiovascular disease, and certain cancers.

Importance of Balance and Moderation

While the anti-inflammatory diet emphasizes certain foods over others, it's important to remember that balance and moderation are key. No single food or nutrient is solely responsible for inflammation or health, and a varied diet that includes a wide range of nutrient-rich foods is essential for overall well-being.

Enjoying occasional treats or indulgences is perfectly acceptable, but they should be consumed in moderation and balanced with healthier choices. By focusing on the big picture of your dietary patterns rather than individual foods, you can create a sustainable eating plan that promotes inflammation reduction and supports long-term health goals.

CHAPTER 3

BUILDING YOUR ANTI-INFLAMMATORY PLATE

Creating nutritious and balanced meals is a cornerstone of the anti-inflammatory diet. By carefully selecting a variety of nutrient-dense foods and paying attention to portion sizes, you can optimize your meals to promote health, reduce inflammation, and support overall well-being.

Creating Balanced Meals

Building a balanced anti-inflammatory plate involves incorporating a combination of macronutrients (carbohydrates, protein, and fat) along with plenty of colorful fruits and vegetables. Here's a guide to help you create balanced meals:

1. Start with non-starchy vegetables: Fill half of your plate with non-starchy vegetables such as leafy greens, broccoli, cauliflower, peppers, and carrots. These vegetables are low in calories and rich in vitamins, minerals, and antioxidants, making them an essential component of a healthy diet.

2. Add lean protein: Include a palm-sized portion of lean protein with each meal. This can include poultry, fish, tofu, tempeh, legumes, or eggs. Protein is important for muscle repair and growth, as well as for keeping you feeling satisfied and full between meals.

3. Incorporate healthy fats: Include a source of healthy fats in your meal, such as avocado, nuts, seeds, or olive oil. Healthy fats are important for brain health, hormone production, and reducing inflammation in the body. Aim to include a thumb-sized portion of healthy fats with each meal.

4. Include whole grains or starchy vegetables: If desired, include a serving of whole grains or starchy vegetables such as quinoa, brown rice, sweet potatoes, or squash. These foods provide energy and fiber, helping to keep you feeling full and satisfied.

5. Add flavor with herbs and spices: Enhance the flavor of your meals with herbs and spices such as turmeric, ginger, garlic, basil, and cilantro. Not only do herbs and spices add delicious flavor to your meals, but many also have anti-inflammatory properties.

6. Stay hydrated: Stay hydrated all day long by drinking lots of water. You can't stay hydrated, digest food properly, or maintain good health without water. Eight glasses of water daily is a good goal to go for, but more is better if you're active or reside in a hotter environment.

Portion Control and Serving Sizes

Portion control is an important aspect of maintaining a healthy weight and preventing overeating. To help you manage your portion amounts, here are some suggestions:

1. Use smaller plates: Using smaller plates can help you control portion sizes by visually reducing the amount of food you serve yourself.

2. Measure portions: Use measuring cups, spoons, or a kitchen scale to measure out appropriate portion sizes of foods such as grains, proteins, and fats.

3. Practice mindful eating: Pay attention to hunger and fullness cues and stop eating when you feel satisfied, rather than continuing to eat until you're uncomfortably full.

4. Eat slowly: Enjoy your meal more fully if you chew it slowly and carefully. Eating more slowly might make you feel full on less food.

5. Be mindful of liquid calories: Be mindful of liquid calories from beverages such as soda, juice, and alcohol, as these can contribute to weight gain without providing a sense of fullness.

Incorporating Variety for Optimal Nutrition

Incorporating a variety of foods into your diet ensures that you're getting a wide range of nutrients to support overall health. Here are some ways for introducing diversity into your meals:

1. Eat the rainbow: Aim to include a variety of colorful fruits and vegetables in your diet, as different colors indicate different nutrients and antioxidants.

2. Try new foods: Be adventurous and try new foods and recipes to keep your meals interesting and diverse.

3. Rotate your protein sources: Rotate your protein sources to include a variety of meats, poultry, fish, legumes, and plant-based proteins such as tofu and tempeh.

4. Experiment with different grains: Experiment with different whole grains such as quinoa, farro, barley, and bulgur to add variety and texture to your meals.

5. Include different cooking methods: Explore different cooking methods such as grilling, roasting, steaming, and sautéing to add variety to your meals and enhance flavor.

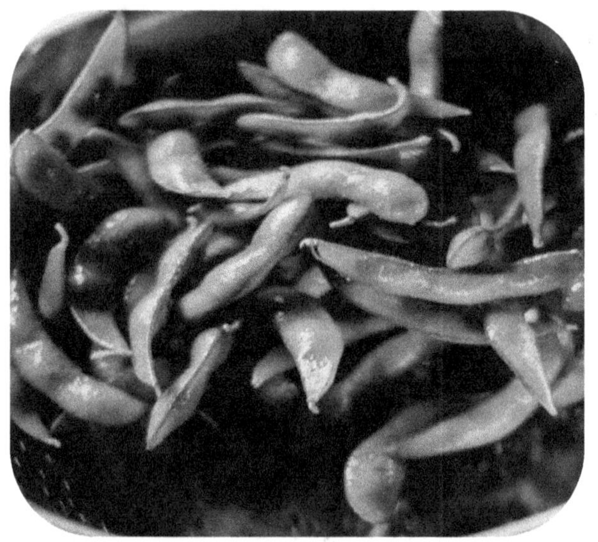

CHAPTER 4:

GROCERY SHOPPING AND MEAL PLANNING

Effective grocery shopping and meal planning are essential components of successfully adopting an anti-inflammatory diet. By stocking your pantry with anti-inflammatory foods, implementing meal planning strategies, and being mindful of budget-friendly shopping techniques, you can simplify the process of eating healthily and sustainably.

Stocking Your Pantry with Anti-Inflammatory Foods

Building a well-stocked pantry is the first step toward creating nutritious and flavorful meals. Here are some key anti-inflammatory foods to include in your pantry:

1. Whole grains: Stock up on whole grains such as quinoa, brown rice, oats, barley, and whole wheat pasta. These grains are rich in fiber and nutrients, providing sustained energy and promoting digestive health.

2. Healthy fats: Keep your pantry stocked with sources of healthy fats such as olive oil, avocado oil, nuts, seeds, and nut butters. These fats are vital for brain function, hormone synthesis, and lowering inflammation in the body.

3. Legumes: Include a variety of legumes such as beans, lentils, chickpeas, and peas in your pantry. Legumes are rich in protein, fiber, and antioxidants, making them a nutritious and versatile addition to soups, salads, and stews.

4. Canned and dried fruits and vegetables: While fresh produce is ideal, canned and dried fruits and vegetables can be convenient options to have on hand for quick and easy meals.

Get products that don't have any artificial sweeteners or preservatives.

5. Herbs and spices: Stock your pantry with a variety of herbs and spices such as turmeric, ginger, garlic, cinnamon, and rosemary. Not only do herbs and spices add flavor to your meals, but many also have potent anti-inflammatory properties.

6. Canned fish: Opt for canned fish such as salmon, sardines, and tuna packed in water or olive oil. These fatty fish are rich in omega-3 fatty acids, which have powerful anti-inflammatory effects.

7. Broths and stocks: Keep broths and stocks on hand for making soups, stews, and sauces. Look for low-sodium options or make your own broth at home for maximum flavor and nutrition.

Meal Planning Strategies

Meal planning is a valuable tool for staying organized, saving time, and making healthier food choices throughout the week. Here are some meal planning techniques to consider:

1. Set aside time for planning: Dedicate a specific time each week to plan your meals for the upcoming week. This could be on a Sunday afternoon or whatever day works best for your schedule.

2. Create a weekly meal plan: Write out a weekly meal plan that includes breakfast, lunch, dinner, and snacks. Consider factors such as your schedule, dietary preferences, and any leftovers or ingredients that need to be used up.

3. Prepare a shopping list: Based on your meal plan, create a shopping list of all the ingredients you'll need for the week. Organize your list by sections of the grocery store to streamline your shopping trip.

4. Batch cook and prep ingredients: Spend some time on meal prep day chopping vegetables, cooking grains, and preparing proteins in advance. This will make it easier to assemble meals throughout the week and reduce the temptation to order takeout on busy nights.

5. Be flexible and adaptable: While it's important to have a plan, it's also important to be flexible and adaptable. Life happens, and there may be times when your meal plan needs to be adjusted. Having a few backup options or quick and easy meals on hand can help.

Tips for Budget-Friendly Shopping

Eating healthily doesn't have to break the bank. With some savvy shopping strategies, you can stick to your budget while still enjoying nutritious and delicious meals. Here are some tips for budget-friendly shopping:

1. Plan your meals around sales and seasonal produce: Take advantage of sales and discounts at your local grocery store by planning your meals around what's on sale. Seasonal produce is often more affordable and flavorful, so base your meals around what's in season.

2. Buy in bulk: Purchase staple items such as grains, beans, nuts, and seeds in bulk to save money in the long run. Many grocery stores offer bulk bins where you can buy as much or as little as you need.

3. Use frozen fruits and vegetables: Frozen fruits and vegetables are often more affordable than fresh and have the added benefit of being convenient and long-lasting. Stock up on frozen produce to use in smoothies, stir-fries, and soups.

4. Opt for generic brands: Consider purchasing generic or store-brand products instead of name brands to save money without sacrificing quality. Compare prices and read labels to ensure you're getting the best value for your money.

5. Limit convenience foods: Pre-packaged and convenience foods are convenient but often come with a higher price tag. Instead, opt for whole foods that require a little more preparation but are more budget-friendly and nutritious in the long run.

By following these strategies for stocking your pantry, meal planning, and budget-friendly shopping, you can make the transition to an anti-inflammatory diet more manageable and sustainable. With a well-stocked pantry, a carefully planned meal schedule, and smart shopping habits, you'll be well-equipped to nourish your body and support your health goals.

CHAPTER 5:

COOKING TECHNIQUES FOR MAXIMUM NUTRITION

Cooking is not just about preparing tasty meals; it's also about preserving the nutritional value of ingredients to support your health and well-being. In this chapter, we'll explore various cooking techniques that maximize nutrition, flavorful seasoning alternatives, and strategies to minimize nutrient loss during food preparation.

Healthy Cooking Methods

1. Steaming: Steaming is a gentle cooking method that preserves the natural flavors and nutrients of foods. Steamed vegetables, fish, and grains retain their texture and color while cooking, making them a nutritious and delicious option.

2. Roasting: often with a drizzle of olive oil and herbs. This cooking method enhances the natural sweetness and flavors of vegetables and produces crispy exteriors while Roasting involves cooking food at high temperatures in the oven retaining moisture and nutrients.

3. Grilling: Grilling is a popular cooking method that adds smoky flavor and charred edges to foods. Choose lean proteins like chicken, fish, or tofu and grill them alongside colorful vegetables for a nutritious and flavorful meal.

4. Stir-frying: Stir-frying involves quickly cooking ingredients in a hot pan with a small amount of oil. This technique preserves the texture and color of vegetables while retaining their nutrients. Use a variety of vegetables, lean proteins, and flavorful sauces for a healthy and satisfying stir-fry.

5. Poaching: Poaching involves cooking food gently in simmering liquid, such as water or broth. This method is ideal for delicate foods like fish, chicken, or eggs, as it preserves their moisture and nutrients while adding subtle flavor.

6. Baking: Baking is a versatile cooking method that can be used to prepare a wide range of nutritious dishes, from whole grain bread to roasted vegetables. Use whole grain flours, natural sweeteners, and healthy fats like olive oil to boost the nutritional value of baked goods.

Flavorful Seasoning Alternatives

1. Herbs and spices: Fresh and dried herbs, as well as spices like turmeric, ginger, garlic, and cinnamon, add flavor and depth to dishes without the need for excessive salt or unhealthy fats.

2. Citrus: Fresh citrus juice and zest, such as lemon, lime, and orange, add brightness and acidity to dishes while enhancing their flavor and nutritional value.

3. Vinegars: Vinegars like balsamic, apple cider, and rice vinegar add tanginess and depth to marinades, dressings, and sauces without added calories or unhealthy additives.

4. Healthy fats: Use heart-healthy fats like olive oil, avocado oil, and nut oils to add richness and flavor to dishes. These fats also contain antioxidants and anti-inflammatory compounds that support overall health.

5. Homemade sauces and dressings: Prepare homemade sauces and dressings using whole food ingredients like

Greek yogurt, tahini, mustard, and herbs for a flavorful and nutritious boost to your meals.

How to Minimize Nutrient Loss

1. Cook foods quickly: Minimize cooking time to reduce nutrient loss. Avoid overcooking vegetables and lean proteins to preserve their vitamins, minerals, and antioxidants.

2. Use minimal water: When cooking vegetables, use minimal water to prevent leaching of water-soluble nutrients like vitamin C and B vitamins. Steaming or microwaving vegetables with a small amount of water is an effective way to retain their nutrients.

3. Store and handle ingredients properly: Store fruits and vegetables in a cool, dark place or the refrigerator to slow down nutrient degradation. Handle ingredients with care to minimize bruising and damage, which can lead to nutrient loss.

4. Eat a variety of foods: Eating a diverse range of foods ensures you receive a wide array of nutrients. Include fruits, vegetables, whole grains, lean meats, and healthy fats into your diet to enhance nutrient intake.

5. Consider raw options: Enjoying some foods raw, such as salads or vegetable crudités, can preserve their natural enzymes and nutrients. Incorporate raw foods into your diet to complement cooked options and maximize nutritional diversity.

CHAPTER 6

Delicious Anti-Inflammatory Recipes Breakfast Ideas Lunch and Dinner Recipes Snacks and Desserts Beverages and Smoothies

Delicious Anti-Inflammatory Recipes

Eating healthily doesn't have to be boring or bland. In fact, with the right ingredients and recipes, you can create delicious and satisfying meals that support your anti-inflammatory goals. In this chapter, we'll explore a variety of mouthwatering recipes designed to nourish your body and tantalize your taste buds.

Breakfast Ideas

1. Turmeric Scrambled Eggs: Whisk together eggs with a pinch of turmeric, black pepper, and chopped spinach. Cook until fluffy and serve with sliced avocado and whole grain toast for a nutrient-rich breakfast.

2. Berry Smoothie Bowl: Blend frozen mixed berries with Greek yogurt, spinach, and a splash of almond milk until smooth. Pour into a bowl and top with sliced bananas, chia seeds, and a drizzle of honey for a refreshing and nutritious start to your day.

3. Quinoa Breakfast Bowl: Cook quinoa according to package instructions and top with sliced almonds, fresh berries, and a dollop of Greek yogurt. Drizzle with honey or maple syrup for added sweetness and enjoy a protein-packed breakfast that will keep you full until lunchtime.

1. Salmon Salad: Grill or bake salmon fillets until cooked through and flaky. Serve over a bed of mixed greens with cherry tomatoes, cucumber slices, and avocado. Drizzle with a lemon-tahini dressing made with tahini, lemon juice, garlic, and olive oil for a flavorful and filling salad.

2. Vegetable Stir-Fry: Stir-fry colorful bell peppers, broccoli, snap peas, and tofu in a wok with a ginger-garlic sauce made from soy sauce, rice vinegar, honey, and sesame oil. A healthy and filling dinner, serve with brown rice or quinoa.

3. Mediterranean Stuffed Bell Peppers: Cut bell peppers in half and remove seeds and membranes. Fill with a mixture of cooked quinoa, chopped tomatoes, olives, feta cheese, and fresh herbs like parsley and oregano. Bake until peppers are tender and filling is heated through for a Mediterranean-inspired dish bursting with flavor.

Snacks and Desserts

1. Greek Yogurt Parfait: Layer Greek yogurt with fresh berries, granola, and a drizzle of honey for a protein-packed snack or dessert that satisfies your sweet tooth while providing a dose of gut-friendly probiotics.

2. Chia Seed Pudding: Mix chia seeds with almond milk, vanilla extract, and a touch of maple syrup. Let sit in the refrigerator for at least an hour to thicken. Serve topped with sliced bananas, chopped nuts, and a sprinkle of cinnamon for a creamy and nutritious treat.

3. Dark Chocolate-Covered Almonds: Melt dark chocolate and dip whole almonds into the melted chocolate. Place on a parchment-lined baking sheet and let cool until chocolate is set. Enjoy as a satisfying snack that provides a dose of antioxidants and healthy fats.

1. Green Smoothie: Blend spinach, kale, pineapple, banana, and coconut water until smooth for a refreshing and nutrient-packed green smoothie that's perfect for breakfast or a post-workout snack.

2. Golden Milk Latte: Warm almond milk with turmeric, ginger, cinnamon, and a touch of honey for a soothing and anti-inflammatory beverage that's ideal for cozy evenings or as a caffeine-free alternative to coffee.

3. Berry Beet Juice: Juice fresh beets, carrots, apples, and ginger for a vibrant and antioxidant-rich beverage that supports detoxification and reduces inflammation. Add a handful of berries for a touch of sweetness and extra flavor.

These recipes are just a starting point for incorporating anti-inflammatory foods into your diet. Feel free to customize them to suit your tastes and preferences, and don't be afraid to experiment with new ingredients and flavors. With a little creativity and a focus on nourishing your body with wholesome foods, you can enjoy delicious meals and support your health and well-being at the same time.

CHAPTER 7

Eating Out and Social Situations Navigating Restaurants with an Anti-Inflammatory Diet Strategies for Dining with Friends and Family Handling Special Occasions and Celebrations

Eating Out and Social Situations

Maintaining an anti-inflammatory diet doesn't mean you have to avoid dining out or socializing with friends and family. With a few strategic approaches and mindful choices, you can still enjoy delicious meals and special occasions while staying true to your health goals. In this chapter, we'll explore tips and strategies for navigating restaurants, dining with loved ones, and handling special occasions with ease.

Navigating Restaurants with an Anti-Inflammatory Diet

1. Research restaurant menus: Before dining out, take some time to research restaurant menus online. Look for restaurants that offer a variety of fresh, whole foods and dishes that can easily be modified to fit your dietary needs.

2. Choose wisely: When dining out, opt for dishes that are based on lean proteins, vegetables, and whole grains. Avoid dishes that are fried, heavily processed, or loaded with added sugars and unhealthy fats.

3. Ask questions: Don't be afraid to ask questions or make special requests when ordering at a restaurant. Ask about ingredient substitutions, cooking methods, and portion sizes to ensure your meal aligns with your dietary preferences and restrictions.

4. Customize your order: Many restaurants are happy to accommodate special dietary needs and preferences. Don't hesitate to ask for modifications to dishes, such as swapping out ingredients or requesting sauces and dressings on the side.

5. Be mindful of portion sizes: Restaurant portions tend to be larger than what you would typically eat at home. Consider sharing a dish with a dining companion or asking for a half portion to avoid overeating.

Strategies for Dining with Friends and Family

1. Communicate your needs: Be open and honest with friends and family about your dietary preferences and restrictions. Let them know in advance if you have any specific dietary concerns or requirements, so they can plan accordingly.

2. Offer to bring a dish: If you're attending a gathering or dinner party, offer to bring a dish that aligns with your dietary needs. This ensures that you'll have at least one option that you can enjoy without worry.

3. Focus on the company: Remember that socializing with loved ones is about more than just the food. Focus on enjoying the conversation, laughter, and connection with friends and family, rather than fixating on what's on your plate.

4. Lead by example: Show your friends and family that eating healthily can be delicious and enjoyable by sharing your favorite recipes and dishes. Lead by example and inspire others to make healthier choices alongside you.

Handling Special Occasions and Celebrations

1. Plan ahead: Anticipate special occasions and plan accordingly by making thoughtful choices about what you'll eat and how you'll indulge. Set realistic goals and boundaries for yourself to ensure that you can enjoy the celebration without feeling guilty or deprived.

2. Focus on balance: Allow yourself to enjoy special treats and indulgences in moderation, but balance them out with healthier choices before and after the celebration. Focus on nourishing your body with nutrient-rich foods and staying active to maintain balance and overall well-being.

3. Practice mindful eating: Pay attention to hunger and fullness cues and eat mindfully during special occasions and celebrations. Take your time to savor each bite, and listen to your body's signals to avoid overeating or feeling uncomfortably full.

4. Stay hydrated: Drink plenty of water throughout the day, especially if you'll be indulging in alcoholic beverages or salty foods during the celebration. Staying hydrated can help prevent overeating and support digestion and overall health.

Remember that maintaining an anti-inflammatory diet is about making sustainable lifestyle choices that support your health and well-being in the long term. By adopting a flexible and mindful approach to eating out and social situations, you can enjoy delicious meals and special occasions while staying on track with your health goals.

CHAPTER 8

Overcoming Challenges and Staying Motivated Dealing with Cravings and Temptations Finding Support and Accountability Celebrating Progress and Milestones

Overcoming Challenges and Staying Motivated

Embarking on any dietary change, including adopting an anti-inflammatory diet, comes with its challenges. From dealing with cravings and temptations to staying motivated in the face of setbacks, this chapter explores strategies for overcoming obstacles and maintaining your commitment to a healthier lifestyle.

Dealing with Cravings and Temptations

1. Understand your triggers: Take note of what triggers your cravings and temptations. Is it stress, boredom, or certain social situations? By identifying your triggers, you can develop strategies to address them more effectively.

2. Practice mindful eating: When cravings strike, pause and ask yourself if you're truly hungry or if you're craving a specific food for emotional reasons. Practice mindful eating by tuning into your body's hunger and fullness signals and choosing nourishing foods that satisfy your cravings in a healthier way.

3. Keep healthy alternatives on hand: Stock your pantry and fridge with healthy alternatives to your favorite indulgences. For example, if you crave something sweet, reach for a piece of fruit or a square of dark chocolate instead of processed sweets.

4. Practice the 80/20 rule: Allow yourself to indulge in your favorite treats occasionally, but aim to make healthy choices 80% of the time. By practicing moderation rather than deprivation, you can satisfy your cravings without derailing your progress.

Finding Support and Accountability

1. Seek out like-minded individuals: Surround yourself with friends, family members, or online communities who share similar health goals and values. It will be fine and awesome if you can have something like a support system.Infact this will provide encouragement, motivation, and accountability on your journey.

2. Enlist a buddy: Partnering up with a friend, family member, or coworker who is also committed to living healthily can increase your chances of success. Hold each other accountable, share successes and challenges, and celebrate milestones together.

3. Join a group or class: Consider joining a support group, wellness program, or fitness class where you can connect with others who are on a similar path. Sharing experiences, tips, and resources with others can help you stay motivated and inspired.

4. Work with a health professional: If you're struggling to stay motivated or overcome obstacles, consider working with a registered dietitian, health coach, or therapist who can provide personalized guidance and support tailored to your individual needs.

1. Set achievable goals: Break your long-term health goals into smaller, more manageable milestones. Celebrate each milestone you reach, whether it's losing a few pounds, sticking to your meal plan for a week, or increasing your physical activity level.

2. Reward yourself: Treat yourself to non-food rewards when you achieve your goals or reach a milestone. This could be anything from a relaxing massage, a new workout outfit, or a weekend getaway to celebrate your progress and hard work.

3. Keep a progress journal: Keep track of your successes, challenges, and progress in a journal or on a digital app. Reflecting on how far you've come can boost your confidence and motivation to continue making positive changes.

4. Celebrate with healthy indulgences: Instead of celebrating milestones with unhealthy treats or indulgences, treat yourself to something that aligns with your health goals. This could be a healthy cooking class, a day of pampering at the spa, or a fun outdoor adventure with friends.

Staying motivated and overcoming challenges is a journey, not a destination. Be patient and kind to yourself, and celebrate every step you take toward living a healthier and more vibrant life. With determination, support, and a positive mindset, you can overcome obstacles and achieve lasting success on your anti-inflammatory journey.

CHAPTER 9

Exercise and Lifestyle Factors the Role of Exercise in Reducing Inflammation Stress Management Techniques Importance of Quality Sleep

Exercise and Lifestyle Factors

In addition to dietary changes, incorporating regular exercise and adopting healthy lifestyle habits are crucial components of an anti-inflammatory lifestyle. This chapter explores the role of exercise in reducing inflammation, effective stress management techniques, and the importance of quality sleep for overall health and well-being.

The Role of Exercise in Reducing Inflammation

1. Promotes circulation: Regular exercise improves blood flow and circulation, which helps deliver oxygen and nutrients to tissues while removing waste products and toxins. This enhanced circulation supports the body's natural anti-inflammatory processes.

2. Reduces oxidative stress: Exercise increases the production of antioxidants in the body, which help neutralize harmful free radicals and reduce oxidative stress. By lowering oxidative stress levels, exercise can help decrease inflammation and protect against chronic diseases.

3. Modulates immune function: Physical activity has been shown to modulate immune function, enhancing the body's ability to fight off infections and reducing the risk of chronic inflammation-related diseases. Regular exercise can help regulate immune responses and promote a healthy balance between pro-inflammatory and anti-inflammatory factors.

4. Supports weight management: Maintaining a healthy weight is important for reducing inflammation, as excess body fat can contribute to chronic low-grade inflammation. Regular exercise helps burn calories, build muscle mass, and improve metabolic function, all of which support weight management and reduce inflammation.

5. Improves insulin sensitivity: Physical activity enhances insulin sensitivity, allowing cells to more effectively uptake glucose from the bloodstream. By improving insulin sensitivity, exercise helps regulate blood sugar levels and reduce inflammation associated with insulin resistance and type 2 diabetes.

Stress Management Techniques

1. Mindfulness meditation: This type of meditation entails paying attention to the here and now while impartially examining thoughts and feelings.

Regular practice can help reduce stress, lower cortisol levels, and promote relaxation and emotional well-being.

2. Deep breathing exercises: Deep breathing exercises, such as diaphragmatic breathing or progressive muscle relaxation, activate the body's relaxation response and help reduce stress and anxiety. Incorporate deep breathing exercises into your daily routine or use them during times of heightened stress.

3. Regular physical activity: Engaging in regular physical activity, such as walking, jogging, swimming, or yoga, can help reduce stress levels and promote a sense of well-being.

Exercise releases endorphins, neurotransmitters that act as natural mood lifters and stress reducers.

4. Healthy lifestyle habits: Prioritize self-care activities such as spending time in nature, practicing hobbies, spending quality time with loved ones

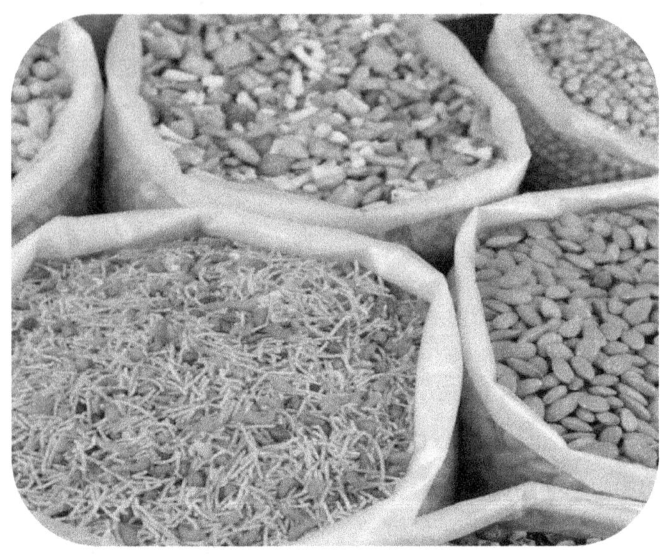

Importance of Quality Sleep

1. Supports immune function: Adequate sleep is essential for maintaining a strong and healthy immune system. During sleep, the body produces cytokines, proteins that help regulate immune responses and protect against infections and inflammation.

2. Regulates inflammation: Sleep plays a critical role in regulating inflammation, with insufficient or poor-quality sleep being associated with higher levels of inflammatory markers in the body. Prioritizing quality sleep can help reduce inflammation and lower the risk of chronic diseases.

3. Promotes tissue repair and regeneration: Sleep is a time for the body to repair and regenerate tissues, including muscles, bones, and organs. During deep sleep stages, growth hormone levels increase, stimulating tissue repair, muscle growth, and overall recovery.

4. Supports cognitive function: Quality sleep is essential for cognitive function, including memory, learning, and problem-solving skills. Adequate rest allows the brain to consolidate memories, process information, and maintain optimal cognitive function throughout the day.

5. Enhances mood and well-being: Sleep plays a vital role in regulating mood and emotional well-being. Chronic sleep deprivation is associated with increased risk of mood disorders such as depression and anxiety, while quality sleep promotes emotional resilience and overall mental health.

Regular exercise, effective stress management techniques, and prioritizing quality sleep are essential components of an anti-inflammatory lifestyle.

CHAPTER 10

Monitoring Progress and Adjusting Your Approach Tracking Symptoms and Dietary Changes When to Reassess and Modify Your Diet Consulting with Healthcare Professionals

Monitoring Progress and Adjusting Your Approach

Successfully following an anti-inflammatory diet involves more than just making initial changes to your eating habits. It requires ongoing monitoring, evaluation, and adjustment to ensure that you're effectively managing inflammation and supporting your overall health. In this chapter, we'll explore strategies for monitoring progress, recognizing when adjustments are needed, and seeking professional guidance when necessary.

Tracking Symptoms and Dietary Changes

1. Keep a food journal: Record your daily food intake, including meals, snacks, and beverages. Note any symptoms you experience, such as digestive issues, joint pain, or fatigue, along with the timing and severity of symptoms. This can help you identify patterns and potential triggers for inflammation.

2. **Monitor changes in symptoms:** Pay attention to changes in your symptoms over time. Are your symptoms improving, worsening, or staying the same? Note any improvements in energy levels, mood, digestion, or other aspects of health, as

well as any lingering or new symptoms that may indicate a need for dietary adjustments.

3. Track dietary changes: Keep track of any changes you make to your diet, including foods you add or eliminate, portion sizes, cooking methods, and meal timing. This can help you identify which dietary changes are having the most significant impact on your symptoms and overall well-being.

When to Reassess and Modify Your Diet

1. Regular reassessment: Schedule regular check-ins with yourself to reassess your progress and evaluate whether your current dietary approach is meeting your needs and goals. Consider reassessing every few weeks or months, depending on your individual health concerns and the severity of your symptoms.

2. Signs that adjustments may be needed: Pay attention to warning signs that indicate your current dietary approach may not be working as well as expected. These signs may include persistent or worsening symptoms, lack of improvement in health outcomes, or difficulty adhering to dietary restrictions.

3. Consult with a healthcare provider: If you're unsure whether your current dietary approach is effective or if you're experiencing persistent or severe symptoms, consider consulting with a healthcare provider, such as a registered dietitian, nutritionist, or integrative medicine specialist. They can help you evaluate your current diet, identify potential areas for improvement, and make personalized recommendations based on your individual needs and health goals.

1. Registered Dietitian/Nutritionist (RDN): A registered dietitian or nutritionist can provide expert guidance on nutrition and dietary strategies for managing inflammation and improving overall health. They can help you develop a personalized anti-inflammatory meal plan, identify potential food sensitivities or intolerances, and offer practical tips for incorporating healthy eating habits into your lifestyle.

2. Integrative Medicine Specialist: An integrative medicine specialist is trained to consider the whole person, including physical, mental, emotional, and spiritual aspects of health. They can help you explore complementary and alternative therapies, such as acupuncture, herbal supplements, or mind-body practices, to support your anti-inflammatory goals.

3. Primary Care Physician: Your primary care physician can provide guidance and oversight of your overall health, including monitoring inflammation markers, managing chronic conditions, and coordinating care with other healthcare providers. They can also refer you to specialists or other healthcare professionals as needed for further evaluation and treatment.

4. Other Specialists: Depending on your specific health concerns and symptoms, you may benefit from consulting with other specialists, such as a gastroenterologist for digestive issues, a rheumatologist for joint pain or autoimmune conditions, or an allergist for food sensitivities or allergies. These specialists can provide additional expertise and treatment options tailored to your individual needs.

Regular monitoring, assessment, and adjustment of your dietary approach are essential for optimizing the effectiveness of an anti-inflammatory diet and promoting long-term health and well-being. By tracking symptoms and dietary changes, knowing when to reassess and modify your diet, and consulting with healthcare professionals when needed, you can take proactive steps to manage inflammation and support your overall health goals.

CONCLUSION

Embarking on the journey of adopting an anti-inflammatory diet is a powerful step towards reclaiming control over your health and well-being. Throughout this guide, we've explored the principles of the anti-inflammatory diet, delved into the science behind inflammation, and provided practical tips for incorporating anti-inflammatory foods into your daily meals.

As you've learned, the anti-inflammatory diet isn't just about what you eat—it's also about how you live. It encompasses lifestyle factors such as regular exercise, stress management, quality sleep, and social support, all of which play crucial roles in reducing inflammation and supporting overall health.

However, it's important to recognize that following an anti-inflammatory diet is not a one-size-fits-all approach. Each person's body is unique, and what works well for one individual may not be the best fit for another. It's essential to listen to your body, pay attention to how different foods and lifestyle factors affect you, and make adjustments as needed to support your individual health goals.

Adopting a healthier way of eating and living is a journey, not a destination. It's normal to encounter challenges along the way, whether it's navigating social situations, managing cravings, or staying motivated. But by staying committed to your goals, seeking support when needed, and celebrating your progress, you can overcome obstacles and create lasting changes that benefit your health and well-being for years to come.

As you continue on your anti-inflammatory journey, be kind to yourself and embrace the process of self-discovery and self-improvement. Celebrate your successes, learn from your setbacks, and keep moving forward with confidence and determination. With dedication, perseverance, and a focus on nourishing your body and mind, you can experience the transformative power of the anti-inflammatory diet and live your life to the fullest.

Here to your health and vitality

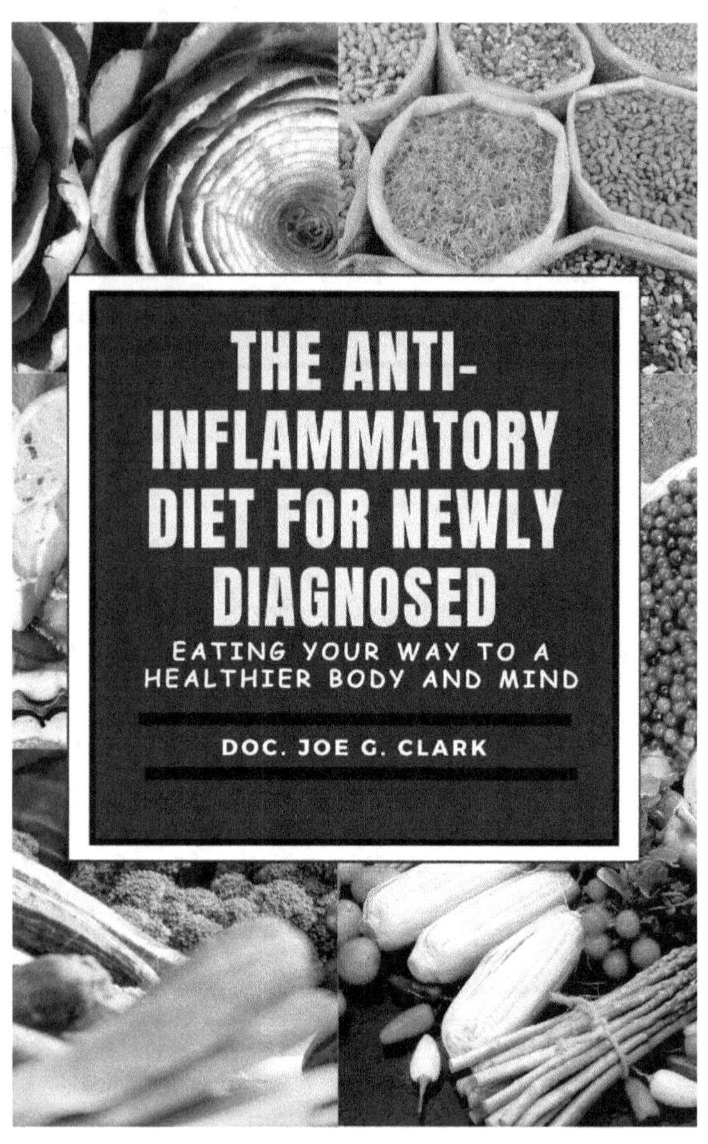

THE ANTI-INFLAMMATORY DIET FOR NEWLY DIAGNOSED
EATING YOUR WAY TO A HEALTHIER BODY AND MIND
DOC. JOE G. CLARK

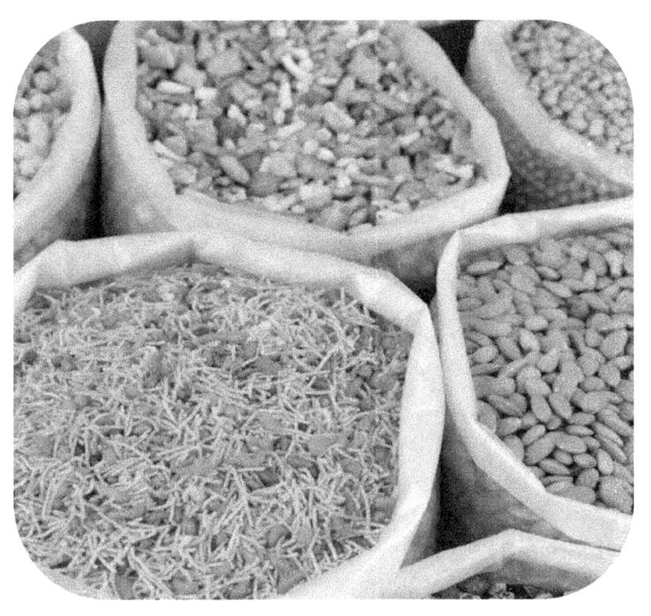